**The Clean Eating**
**101 Amazing Whole Fo**
**Casserole, Slow Cooker a**
**Inspired by The Medi**

CW01582083

by **Alissa Noel Grey**

# Table Of Contents

## Would you like to lose weight? Tone up? Feel healthier and have more energy?

Clean Eating is a healthy way of life to learn and follow; it is not a fad diet. Clean Eating is easy and common sense and it will make you feel energized and happy in no time at all. Eating whole natural food will become your second nature to you once you realize you can throw together a healthy dinner in the same amount of time you'd need to order a takeout.

Clean Eating is so amazing because it is simply about eating more of the best and healthiest options in each of the food groups - and eating less of the not-so-healthy ones. In our world where food is full of frightening artificial additives and ingredients, clean eating is a very straight-forward and easy way to adopt a healthy lifestyle. There is overwhelming evidence that a diet rich in local fruit, vegetables, lean meats and meatless proteins, such as lentils, beans or chickpeas, whole grains, nuts and seeds is very good for our overall health. And while there may be more than one right way to eat, all scientists agree on one thing – the more real, natural, unprocessed food you eat, the better. Since you don’t have to count calories or give up your favorite food, clean eating is deceptively simple. Clean eating and the Mediterranean diet have a lot in common. A fundamental characteristic of the Mediterranean diet is that food is cooked using easily available ingredients - local, whole food products that we can buy around the corner or grow in our own backyard. All my recipes inspired by the Mediterranean diet are easy and healthy because they include good fats like olive and avocado oils, fresh vegetables, protein-rich legumes, lean meats, whole grains, and aromatic, superfood herbs and spices.

Following a clean eating plan is much easier than you might think. It doesn't require a lot of extra time or money to eat fresh local produce and the only rigid rule you must follow is to avoid highly processed foods that contain refined white sugars and refined white flours, excessive salt, preservatives, additives, artificial sweeteners and trans fats. So if you learn to skip most packaged and processed foods and read labels to avoid added sugars, salts, and fats, you have started your journey to a better you.

# Clean Eating Salad and Side Dish Recipes

## Chicken and Potato Salad with Olives

**Serves: 4-5**

**Prep time: 5 min**

**Ingredients:**

1 lb chicken breast halves, cooked and sliced

1 lb boiled potatoes, peeled and diced

1/2 red onion, chopped

1/4 cup black olives, pitted

1 tbsp capers

1/2 tsp ground ginger

1 tsp cumin

1 tsp paprika

1/4 tsp dried oregano

1/2 tsp salt

1/4 tsp black pepper

3 tbsp lemon juice

4 tbsp extra virgin olive oil

1/4 cup parsley leaves, chopped

**Directions:**

In a small glass bowl, whisk together the lemon juice, cumin, paprika, salt, black pepper, ginger, and oregano. Whisk in 4 tablespoons of the olive oil.

In a salad bowl, combine the warm potatoes with half of the dressing. Add in the sliced chicken, onion, olives, capers, parsley, and the remaining dressing, and toss to combine.

## Simple Greek Chicken Salad

**Serves: 4-5**

**Prep time: 5 min**

**Ingredients:**

3 chicken breast halves, cooked and sliced

1 small cucumber, sliced

2 medium tomatoes, sliced

1/2 red onion, sliced

1/4 cup black olives, pitted

1 cup crumbled feta cheese

1 tsp dried oregano

1 tbsp lemon juice

2 tbsp extra virgin olive oil

1/4 cup parsley leaves, finely cut

salt, to taste

**Directions:**

Place the chicken, tomatoes, cucumber, red onion, olives, feta, and parsley in a salad bowl.

Toss to combine, drizzle with lemon juice and olive oil, sprinkle with oregano, toss again, and serve.

## Mediterranean Chicken and Pasta Salad

**Serves: 5-6**

**Prep time: 5 min**

**Ingredients:**

3 cups small pasta, cooked

3 chicken breast halves, cooked and shredded

1 cup cherry tomatoes, halved

1 yellow bell pepper, sliced

1 small red onion, finely cut

1/2 cup black olives, pitted

1 tbsp capers

1/3 cup pine nuts, toasted

7-8 fresh basil leaves, finely chopped

**for the dressing:**

3 tbsp lemon juice

3 tbsp extra virgin olive oil

2 garlic cloves, crushed

salt, to taste

**Directions:**

Place pasta, chicken, tomatoes, bell pepper, red onion, basil, olives, capers and pine nuts in a large bowl.

Prepare the dressing by whisking lemon juice, olive oil, garlic, and salt. Pour the dressing over the salad, toss to combine, and serve.

## Moroccan Tomato Salad

**Serves: 4-5**

**Prep time: 5 min**

**Ingredients:**

2 lbs ripe tomatoes, peeled and diced

1 celery rib, diced

1 red onion, finely cut

1 green bell pepper, finely cut

2 tbsp capers

1 tsp dried mint

1 tbsp grated lemon peel

2 tbsp lemon juice

3 tbsp extra virgin olive oil

salt and black pepper, to taste

**Directions:**

In a deep salad bowl, toss the tomatoes with the celery, onion, green bell pepper, lemon peel and capers.

Season with dried mint, salt and black pepper to taste. Drizzle with lemon juice and olive oil and toss to combine. Refrigerate for at least 30 minutes before serving.

## Warm Tomato Salad

**Serves: 4-5**

**Prep time: 10 min**

**Ingredients:**

4 tomatoes, sliced

1 cup cherry tomatoes, halved

½ small red onion, very finely cut

2 garlic cloves, crushed

1 tbsp dried parsley

2 tbsp extra virgin olive oil

1 tbsp balsamic vinegar

**Directions:**

Gently heat oil in a non-stick frying pan over low heat. Cook garlic and tomatoes, stirring occasionally, for 4-5 minutes or until tomatoes are warm but firm.

Remove from heat and place in a plate. Add in red onion, vinegar and dried parsley. Season with salt and pepper to taste and serve.

## Roasted Garlicky Peppers

**Serves 4-6**

**Prep time: 15 min**

**Ingredients:**

2 lbs red and green bell peppers

3-4 cloves garlic, chopped

1/2 cup fresh parsley, finely cut

4-5 tbsp extra virgin oil

4 tbsp white wine vinegar

salt and pepper, to taste

**Directions:**

Roast the peppers in the oven at 480 F until the skins are a little burnt. Place them in a brown paper bag or a lidded container and leave them covered for about 10 minutes. Peel the skins and remove the seeds.

Cut the peppers into 1 inch strips lengthwise and layer them in a salad bowl. Mix together the oil, vinegar, salt and pepper, chopped garlic and the chopped parsley leaves. Pour over the peppers. Serve chilled.

## Mediterranean Beef Salad

**Serves: 4-5**

**Prep time: 5 min**

**Ingredients:**

8 oz quality roast beef, thinly sliced

1 avocado, peeled and diced

2 tomatoes, diced

1 cucumber, peeled and diced

1 yellow pepper, sliced

1 carrot, shredded

1 cup black olives, pitted and halved

2-3 fresh basil leaves, torn

2-3 fresh oregano leaves

1 tbsp balsamic vinegar

4 tbsp extra virgin olive oil

salt and black pepper, to taste

**Directions:**

Combine the avocado and all vegetables in a large salad bowl. Add in basil and oregano leaves.

Season with salt and pepper, drizzle with balsamic vinegar and olive oil, and toss to combine. Top with roast beef and serve.

## Ground Beef Salad with Creamy Avocado Dressing

**Serves: 4-5**

**Prep time: 10 min**

**Ingredients:**

1 green lettuce, cut in stripes

2-3 green onions, finely cut

1 garlic clove, crushed

½ cup black olives, pitted and halved

4-5 radishes, sliced

8 oz ground beef

1/2 tsp cumin

1/2 tsp dried oregano

1 tsp paprika

2 tbsp extra virgin olive oil

salt and pepper, to taste

**for the dressing:**

1 avocado, peeled and cut

1 tbsp extra virgin olive oil

4 tbsp lemon juice

1 garlic clove

1 tbsp water

1/2 tsp salt

**Directions:**

Blend the dressing ingredients until smooth.

Heat olive oil in a medium saucepan and gently cook the ground beef and the seasonings, stirring, for 5-6 minutes, or until cooked through.

Place the lettuce, cooked beef and all other salad ingredients in a bowl. Toss well to combine. Drizzle with dressing and serve.

## Tuna and Lettuce Salad

**Serves: 4**

**Prep time: 5 min**

**Ingredients:**

1 head green lettuce, washed cut in thin strips

1 cup chopped watercress

1 cucumber, peeled and chopped

1 tomato, diced

1 can water-packed tuna, drained and broken into small chunks

7-8 radishes, sliced

3-4 spring onions, chopped

juice of half lemon

3 tbsp extra virgin olive oil

**Directions:**

Mix all the vegetables in a large bowl. Add the tuna and season with lemon juice, olive oil and salt to taste.

## Easy Bean and Tuna Salad

**Serves: 4**

**Prep time: 5 min**

**Ingredients:**

1 cup cooked white beans, drained

1 can water-packed tuna, broken into chunks

1/2 red onion, chopped

1/2 cup fresh parsley leaves, chopped

1 tsp dried mint

salt and black pepper, to taste

juice of one lemon

3 tbsp extra virgin olive oil

**Directions:**

Put tuna chunks and beans in a salad bowl and toss to combine. Add in onions, parsley, mint, lemon juice and olive oil, and toss to combine.

Season with salt and black pepper to taste. Serve chilled.

## Clean Eating Tuna Salad

**Serves: 4**

**Prep time: 5 min**

**Ingredients:**

2 cans water-packed tuna, broken into chunks

1 red onion, chopped

2 tomatoes, diced

2 hard boiled eggs, diced

1 tbsp pesto

3 tbsp lemon juice

3 tbsp olive oil

salt and black pepper, to taste

**Directions:**

Put tune, tomatoes, eggs, and onion in a salad bowl and toss to combine.

Whisk the pesto with lemon juice and olive oil. Season with salt and black pepper to taste, and drizzle over the salad. Serve chilled.

## Spinach with Steamed Beets and Feta Cheese

**Serves: 4-5**

**Prep time: 15 min**

**Ingredients:**

3 medium beets, steamed, peeled and diced

1 bag baby spinach leaves

1/2 cup walnuts, toasted

4 oz feta, crumbled

4-5 spring onions, chopped

**for the dressing:**

1 garlic clove, crushed

2 tbsp extra virgin olive oil

2 tbsp lemon juice

1 tbsp finely cut dill

**Directions:**

Wash the beets, steam, peel and dice them. Arrange the spinach leaves in a large salad bowl. Scatter the beets, onions, walnuts, and feta over the spinach.

In a smaller bowl or cup, combine the oil, lemon juice, garlic and dill. Whisk until smooth, season with salt and pepper, and drizzle over the salad.

## Mediterranean Spinach Salad with Yogurt

**Serves: 4**

**Prep time: 5 min**

**Ingredients:**

1 bag baby spinach

4-5 spring onions, finely chopped

1 cucumber, peeled and cut

1/2 cup walnuts, halved and roasted

1/3 cup Greek yogurt

2 tbsp red wine vinegar

3 tbsp extra virgin olive oil

salt and black pepper, to taste

**Directions:**

Whisk yogurt, olive oil and vinegar in a small bowl.

Place the baby spinach leaves in a large salad bowl. Add the onions, cucumber and walnuts. Season with black pepper and salt, stir, and toss with the dressing.

## Feta Cheese Stuffed Tomatoes

**Serves 4**

**Prep time: 5 min**

**Ingredients:**

4 large ripe tomatoes

2 cups feta cheese, crumbled

1 cup finely cut parsley

1 tsp paprika

2 tbsp extra virgin olive oil

**Directions:**

Cut the top of each tomato in such a way as to be able to stuff the tomato and cover with the cap. Scoop out the seeds and central part of the tomatoes to create a hollow.

Mash the scooped out tomato parts with a fork, add to the feta cheese and stir to make a homogeneous mixture. Add in the olive oil, paprika and parsley. Stuff the tomatoes with the cheese mixture and cover with the caps. Serve chilled.

## Moroccan Carrot Salad with Oranges and Dates

**Serves: 4**

**Prep time: 10 min**

**Ingredients:**

4 carrots, shredded

3 oranges, peeled and cut

1 orange zested and juiced

1 lemon, zested and juiced

1/2 lb dates, pitted and thinly sliced lengthwise

1 tsp cumin

1/4 tsp cinnamon

1 tbsp honey

2 tbsp extra virgin olive oil

salt and pepper, to taste

**Directions:**

In a bowl, whisk the orange and lemon juice with the orange and lemon zests, honey, cinnamon and cumin. Gradually add in the olive oil and season with salt. Add in the dates and toss to combine.

Using a very sharp knife, peel the oranges, carefully removing all of the bitter white pith. Cutting in between the membranes, release the orange sections into the bowl with the dressing.

Arrange the shredded carrots on a platter, spoon the oranges and dates around it and drizzle with the dressing.

## Beet Salad with Walnuts

**Serves: 4**

**Prep time: 25 min**

**Ingredients:**

3 medium beets, steamed and diced

1 red onion, sliced

1/2 cup walnuts, halved

1 cup strained Greek yogurt

1 tbsp lemon juice

2 tbsp olive oil

4-5 mint leaves, chopped

½ tsp salt

**Directions:**

Wash the beets, trim the stems, and steam them over boiling water until cooked through.

Dice the beets and place them in a salad bowl. Add in walnuts and onion and toss to combine. Sprinkle with fresh mint leaves.

Whisk the yogurt with garlic, olive oil and lemon juice until smooth. Pour over the diced beets and toss to combine. Serve chilled.

## Warm Beet and Lentil Salad

**Serves: 5-6**

**Prep time: 10 min**

**Ingredients:**

1 cup cooked brown lentils, drained

1 cup boiled or steamed beets, diced

1 cup baby arugula leaves

1 small red onion, chopped

2 garlic cloves, crushed

6 oz feta cheese, crumbled

1 tbsp extra virgin olive oil

**for the dressing**

3 tbsp extra virgin olive oil

1 tbsp red wine vinegar

1 tsp summer savory

salt and black pepper, to taste

**Directions:**

Heat a tablespoon of olive oil in a skillet and gently sauté the onion for 2-3 minutes or until softened. Add in garlic, lentils and beets. Cook, stirring, for 2 minutes.

Whisk together the remaining olive oil, vinegar, summer savory, salt and pepper. Add to the lentils and toss to coat. Combine baby arugula, feta and lentil mixture in a bowl. Toss gently to combine and serve.

## Roasted Vegetables with Yogurt Dressing

**Serves: 4-5**

**Prep time: 30 min**

**Ingredients:**

3 tomatoes, halved

1 zucchini, quartered

1 fennel bulb, thinly sliced

2 small eggplants, ends trimmed, quartered

1 large red pepper, halved, deseeded, cut into strips

2 medium onions, quartered

1 tsp oregano

2 tbsp extra virgin olive oil

**for the dressing**

2/3 cup Greek yogurt

1 tbsp fresh lemon juice

1 small garlic clove, chopped

**Directions:**

Place the zucchini, eggplant, pepper, fennel, onions, tomatoes and olive oil on a lined baking sheet. Season with salt, pepper and oregano and roast in a 500 F oven until golden, about 20 minutes.

Whisk the yogurt, lemon juice and garlic in a bowl. Taste and season with salt and pepper. Divide the vegetables in 4-5 plates. Top with the yogurt mixture and serve.

## Mediterranean Avocado Salad

**Serves: 5-6**

**Prep time: 10 min**

**Ingredients:**

2 avocados, peeled, halved and cut into cubes

1 ciabatta roll, cut into small cubes

2 cups cherry tomatoes, halved

½ red onion, thinly sliced

1 large cucumber, peeled, halved, sliced

½ cup green olives, pitted, halved

½ cup black olives, pitted, sliced

6 oz feta cheese, cut into cubes

7-8 fresh basil leaves, torn

½ cup parsley leaves, finely cut

1 tsp dried oregano

4 tbsp extra virgin olive oil

3 tbsp red wine vinegar

**Directions:**

Line a baking tray with baking paper and place ciabatta cubes. Drizzle with one tablespoon of olive oil. Season with salt and pepper and sprinkle with oregano. Gently toss to coat and cook under the grill for 2-3 minutes or until golden. Set aside to cool.

Place all vegetables, feta, basil, olives, and ciabatta cubes in a large salad bowl. Gently toss to combine then sprinkle with vinegar and remaining olive oil. Season with salt and pepper and toss again. Sprinkle with parsley and serve.

## Granny's Favorite Couscous Salad

**Serves: 4**

**Prep time: 15 min**

**Ingredients:**

1 cup medium couscous

11/2 cup hot water

3 ripe tomatoes, diced

1/2 cup black olives, pitted and chopped

5 green onions, finely chopped

4 tbsp extra virgin olive oil

4 tbsp lemon juice

1 tbsp dry mint

2-3 fresh mint leaves

salt, to taste

**Directions:**

Place the couscous in a large bowl and pour over a cup and a half of boiling water. Stir, cover, and set aside for 10 minutes. Fluff with a fork and stir in the tomatoes, olives and onions.

In a small bowl, whisk olive oil, lemon juice, dried mint, fresh mint and salt. Pour over the couscous salad, stir until well combined and serve.

## Warm Leek and Sweet Potato Salad

**Serves 4-5**

**Prep time: 30 min**

**Ingredients:**

1.5 lb sweet potato, unpeeled, cut into 1 inch pieces

4 small leeks, trimmed and cut into 1 inch slices

5-6 white mushrooms, halved

1 cup baby arugula leaves

2 tbsp extra virgin olive oil

**for the dressing**

½ cup Greek yogurt

1 tbsp Dijon mustard

**Directions:**

Preheat oven to 350 F. Line a baking tray with baking paper. Place the sweet potato, leeks and mushrooms on the baking tray. Drizzle with olive oil and toss to coat. Roast for 20 minutes or until golden.

Combine yogurt and mustard in a small bowl or cup. Place the roasted vegetables in a salad bowl, drizzle with the yogurt mixture and top with arugula leaves.

## Roasted Sweet Potato and Quinoa Salad

**Serves: 5-6**

**Prep time: 15 min**

**Ingredients:**

1 cup cooked quinoa

2 lb sweet potatoes, peeled

1/2 cup roasted walnuts

1 cup beet, lentil or mixed sprouts

3-4 fresh basil leaves

2 tbsp extra virgin olive oil

2 tbsp balsamic vinegar

salt, to taste

**Directions:**

Cut the sweet potatoes into chunks and arrange on a baking sheet sprinkled with cinnamon, olive oil and a little salt and black pepper. Toss to coat well.

Bake at 350 F for 15 minutes, or until golden and crisp.

In a salad bowl, combine quinoa, sweet potatoes, sprouts and walnuts. Drizzle with balsamic vinegar and olive oil and serve.

## Homemade Hummus

**Serves: 5-6**

**Prep time: 5 min**

**Ingredients:**

1 15 oz can chickpeas, drained, (Note: Opt for BPA-free cans)

1/3 cup tahini

3 tbsp extra virgin olive oil

½ lemon, juiced

2-3 small garlic cloves, chopped

1-2 tsp cumin, or to taste

1 tsp salt

water

1 tbsp extra virgin olive oil, to serve

1 tbsp finely cut parsley, to serve

1 tsp paprika, to serve

**Directions:**

Drain the chickpeas and if possible, remove the skins. Place the chickpeas in the blender and pulse. Add the tahini, lemon juice, garlic, olive oil, cumin and salt, and blend until smooth, gradually adding the water to the mix until the mixture is completely smooth.

To serve, top with olive oil, parsley, and sprinkle with paprika.

## Zucchini and Avocado Dip

**Serves: 4**

**Prep time: 5 min**

**Ingredients:**

1 large zucchini, peeled and diced

1 avocado, peeled and chopped

2 garlic cloves, chopped

2 tbsp tahini

2 tbsp extra virgin olive oil

1/4 cup lemon juice

1 tsp cumin

salt, to taste

**Directions:**

Combine all ingredients in a blender and pulse until smooth.

Serve with crackers, fresh vegetables or chips.

# Clean Eating Soup Recipes

## Healthy Chicken and Oat Soup

**Serves: 4**

**Prep time: 35 min**

**Ingredients:**

3 chicken breasts, diced

1 small onion, chopped

3 garlic cloves

1 large carrot, chopped

1 red or green pepper, chopped

1 celery rib, chopped

1/2 cup quick-cooking oats

5 cups water

1 bay leaf

1 tsp salt

1/2 cup fresh parsley leaves, finely cut

black pepper, to taste

lemon juice, to serve

**Directions:**

Place the chicken, bay leaf, celery, carrot, onion, red pepper, water, and salt into a pot.

Bring to the boil, reduce heat, and simmer for 30 minutes. Discard the bay leaf, season with salt and pepper, add in the oats and parsley, simmer for 5 more minutes, and serve sprinkled with lemon juice.

## Moroccan Chicken Soup

**Serves: 4-5**

**Prep time: 30 min**

**Ingredients:**

3-4 skinless, boneless chicken thighs, cut into bite-sized pieces

1 onion, finely cut

2 garlic cloves, chopped

1 small zucchini, peeled and diced

1 cup butternut squash, peeled and cut in 1/2-inch pieces

2 tbsp tomato paste

5 cups water

1/3 cup uncooked couscous

1/2 tsp cumin

1/4 teaspoon ground cinnamon

1 tbsp paprika

1 tbsp dried basil

2 tbsp orange zest

3 tbsp extra virgin olive oil

**Directions:**

Heat olive oil in a soup pot over medium heat. Gently sauté onion, for 1 minute, stirring. Add in garlic, basil and chicken, and cook for 2-3 minutes, or until the chicken is sealed.

Stir in cumin, cinnamon and paprika. Add butternut squash and stir again. Dissolve the tomato paste in the water and add to the soup.

Bring to a boil, reduce heat and simmer for 10-15 minutes.

Stir in couscous, salt, and the zucchini and cook until the butternut squash is tender.

Remove from heat, season with salt and pepper to taste, stir in the orange rind, and serve.

## Mediterranean Chicken Soup

**Serves: 4-5**

**Prep time: 35 min**

**Ingredients:**

3 chicken breast halves

2 carrots, chopped

1 celery stalk, chopped

1 small onion, chopped

1/3 cup rice

6 cups water

1/2 cup olives, pitted and halved

salt and black pepper, to taste

1/2 cup fresh coriander, finely cut, to serve

lemon juice, to serve

**Directions:**

Place the chicken breasts in a soup pot together with the onion, carrots, celery, salt, black pepper and water.

Bring to a boil, add in rice and olives, stir, and reduce heat. Simmer for 30-35 minutes then remove the chicken from the pot and let it cool slightly.

Shred the chicken and return it back to the pot. Stir, and serve sprinkled with fresh coriander and lemon juice.

## Greek Chicken Soup

**Serves: 4**

**Prep time: 35 min**

**Ingredients:**

3 chicken breast halves, diced

1/3 cup rice

4 cups water

1 small onion, finely cut

3 egg yolks

1/2 cup fresh lemon juice

3 tbsp extra virgin olive oil

1 tsp salt

1/2 tsp black pepper

1/2 cup fresh parsley, finely cut, to serve

**Directions:**

In a soup pot, heat the olive oil and gently sauté the onion until translucent. Add in the water and bring to a boil.

Stir in the rice and the chicken, reduce heat, and simmer until the rice is almost done.

Whisk the egg yolks and lemon juice together in a small bowl. Gently add this mixture to the soup whisking constantly. Do not boil any more. Season with salt and pepper, and garnish with finely chopped parsley. Serve hot.

## Bean, Chicken and Bacon Soup

**Serves 4-5**

**Prep time: 50 min**

**Ingredients:**

2-3 bacon strips, cut

2 cups cooked and diced chicken

1/4 cup dried kidney beans, soaked overnight

1 small onion, chopped

2 garlic cloves, chopped

4 cups water

3 ripe tomatoes, diced

1 bay leaf

1/2 tsp dried oregano

1/2 tsp dried basil

salt and pepper, to taste

**Directions:**

In a deep soup pot, gently cook the onion and bacon, stirring, for 3-4 minutes. Add in the garlic and cook until just fragrant.

Add in the water, tomatoes, beans and seasonings and bring to a boil. Cover, reduce heat, and simmer for 40 minutes. Add in the chicken and simmer for 5 minutes more.

## Easy Chicken Vermicelli Soup

**Serves 4**

**Prep time: 40 min**

**Ingredients:**

3 chicken breast halves

1/2 onion, finely cut

1 garlic clove, chopped

1/2 cup vermicelli

1 carrot, grated

4 cups water

1 tsp salt

1/2 tsp black pepper

1 egg, beaten

2 tbsp lemon juice

**Directions:**

Place the chicken breasts and the onion in a soup pot together with 4 cups of water. Add in one teaspoon of salt and bring to a boil.

Cook for 30 minutes or until the chicken is cooked through. Take the chicken out of the pot, let it cool a little, dice it, and put it back in the soup.

Stir in the carrot, garlic and vermicelli. Reduce heat and simmer over medium heat for 5 minutes.

Whisk the egg and lemon juice in a bowl and slowly stir this mixture into the soup. Do not boil again.

## Spanish Cold Prawn Soup

**Serves 4-5**

**Prep time: 20 min**

**Ingredients:**

2 lbs cooked, peeled and deveined prawn

2 cups tomato juice

2 cups prawn stock

3 spring onions, chopped

2 avocados, peeled and diced

1 cucumber, peeled and diced

2 large tomatoes, diced

1 cup finely chopped parsley

2 tbsp lime juice

salt and pepper, to taste

**Directions:**

Combine the tomato juice and prawn stock. Stir in the prawns, avocados, cucumber, tomatoes, spring onions, parsley, lime juice, salt and pepper.

Refrigerate until ready to serve.

## Mediterranean Fish and Quinoa Soup

**Serves: 4-5**

**Prep time: 30 min**

**Ingredients:**

1 lb cod fillets, cubed

1 onion, chopped

3 tomatoes, chopped

1/2 cup quinoa, rinsed

1 red pepper, chopped

1 carrot, chopped

1/2 cup black olives, pitted and sliced

1 garlic clove, crushed

a pinch of cayenne pepper

1 bay leaf

1 tsp dried thyme

1 tsp dried dill

½ tsp black pepper

½ cup white wine

4 cups water

3 tbsp extra virgin olive oil

salt and black pepper, to taste

1/2 cup fresh parsley, finely cut

**Directions:**

Heat the olive oil over medium heat and sauté the onion, red pepper, garlic and carrot until tender.

Stir in the cayenne pepper, bay leaf, herbs, salt and pepper. Add in the white wine, water, quinoa and tomatoes and bring to a boil.

Reduce heat, cover, and cook for 10 minutes. Stir in the olives and fish and cook for another 10 minutes. Stir in parsley and serve hot.

## Fish and Pasta Soup

**Serves: 4-5**

**Prep time: 15 min**

**Ingredients:**

3 white fish fillets, cut into strips

2 carrots, cut into ribbons

1 small zucchini, peeled and cut into ribbons

5-6 white button mushrooms, sliced

1 celery stalk, finely cut

1 cup baby spinach

7 oz small pasta

5 cups water

3 tbsp soy sauce

1 tsp ground ginger

salt and black pepper, to taste

**Directions:**

Place water and soy sauce in a deep soup pot. Bring to a boil and add in pasta, carrots, celery, zucchini, mushrooms and ginger.

Simmer, partially covered, for 10 minutes then add in the fish and simmer for 5 minutes more or until the fish is cooked through.

Stir in the spinach and cook until it wilts. Season with black pepper and salt to taste and serve.

## Homemade Meatball Soup

**Serves 4-5**

**Prep time: 30 min**

**Ingredients:**

1 lb ground beef

1 small onion, grated

1 onion, chopped

1 egg, lightly beaten

2 garlic cloves, crushed

1 cup baby spinach, coarsely chopped

4-5 fresh basil leaves, finely chopped

1 cup tomato sauce

3 cups homemade beef broth

2 tbsp extra virgin olive oil

salt and black pepper, to taste

**Directions:**

Combine ground beef, onion, garlic, and egg in a large bowl. Season with salt and pepper to taste. Mix well with hands and roll teaspoonfuls of the mixture into balls. Place meatballs on a large plate.

Heat olive oil into a large deep saucepan and sauté the onion and garlic until transparent. Add in the tomato sauce and broth and bring to a boil over high heat. Stir in the meatballs.

Reduce heat to medium-low and simmer, uncovered, for 20 minutes. Add in spinach, basil, salt and pepper and simmer, uncovered, until the spinach wilts, about 1 minute.

## Split Pea Soup with Ham and Barley

**Serves: 4-5**

**Prep time: 35 min**

**Ingredients:**

3/4 cup dry yellow split peas

2 carrots, chopped

1/2 lb low-sodium, nitrate-free, lean cooked ham, cut into 1/2-inch cubes

1 zucchini, peeled and diced

1 potato, peeled and diced

1 cup quick-cooking pearl barley

2 tsp dried sage

4 cups water

4 tbsp extra virgin olive oil

salt and black pepper, to taste

**Directions:**

In a medium pot, bring 2 cups water to a boil on high heat. Add split peas and reduce heat to medium-low. Simmer, uncovered, for 20 minutes. Drain and set aside.

Gently heat olive oil in a large soup pot. Add in onions, carrot and ham and cook for 1-2 minutes, stirring, until vegetables are tender.

Add in zucchini, sage, barley and water. Season to taste with salt and pepper and simmer for 15 minutes.

## Creamy Brussels Sprouts Soup

**Serves: 4-5**

**Prep time: 30 min**

**Ingredients:**

1 lb frozen Brussels sprouts

2 potatoes, peeled and chopped

1 large onion, chopped

3 garlic cloves, minced

4 cups water

3 tbsp extra virgin olive oil

1/2 tsp curry powder

salt and black pepper, to taste

**Directions:**

Gently heat olive oil in a large saucepan over medium-high heat. Cook the onion and garlic and for 3-4 minutes until tender. Add in Brussels sprouts, potato, curry and water.

Cover and bring to a boil, then reduce heat and simmer for 20 minutes, stirring from time to time. Remove from heat and blend until smooth. Return to pan and cook until heated through.

## Creamy Potato Soup

**Serves: 4-5**

**Prep time: 35 min**

**Ingredients:**

6 medium potatoes, cut into small cubes

1 leek, white part only, chopped

1 carrot, chopped

1 zucchini, peeled and chopped

1 celery stalk, chopped

3 cups water

1 cup milk

3 tbsp extra virgin olive oil

salt and black pepper, to taste

**Directions:**

Gently heat olive oil in a deep saucepan and sauté the onion for 2-3 minutes. Add in potatoes, carrot, zucchini and celery and cook for 2-3 minutes, stirring.

Add water and salt and bring to a boil, then lower heat and simmer until the vegetables are tender. Blend until smooth, add milk, blend some more and serve.

## Leek, Brown Rice and Potato Soup

**Serves: 4-5**

**Prep time: 35 min**

**Ingredients:**

3 potatoes, peeled and diced

2 leeks, finely chopped

1/4 cup brown rice

5 cups water

3 tbsp extra virgin olive oil

lemon juice, to taste

**Directions:**

Heat olive oil in a deep soup pot and sauté leeks for 3-4 minutes. Add in potatoes and cook for a minute more. Stir in water, bring to a boil, and add the brown rice.

Reduce heat and simmer for 30 minutes. Add lemon juice, to taste, and serve.

## Mediterranean Chickpea Soup

**Serves: 5-6**

**Prep time: 30 min**

**Ingredients:**

1 can chickpeas, drained and rinsed (Note: Opt for BPA-free cans)

1 small onion, chopped

2 garlic cloves, minced

3 ripe tomatoes, diced

3 cups water

1 cup milk

2 bay leaves

1/2 tsp dried oregano

3 tbsp extra virgin olive oil

**Directions:**

Heat olive oil in a deep soup pot and sauté the onion and garlic for 1-2 minutes. Add in water, chickpeas, tomatoes, bay leaves, and oregano.

Bring the soup to a boil then reduce heat and simmer for 20 minutes. Add in milk and cook for 1-2 minutes more.

Set aside to cool, discard the bay leaves and blend until smooth.

## Crock Pot Tomato Basil Soup

**Serves: 5-6**

**Prep time: 3 min**

**Cooking time: 5-6 hours**

**Ingredients:**

5-6 ripe tomatoes diced

1/3 cup rice

3 cups water

1 large onion, diced

4 garlic cloves, minced

1 tsp salt

1 tbsp dried basil

1 tsp paprika

1 tsp sugar

3 tbsp extra virgin olive oil

½ bunch fresh parsley, to serve

**Directions:**

In a skillet, gently sauté the onion and garlic for 2-3 minutes or until transparent. Add them together with all other ingredients to the slow cooker.

Cook on low for 5-7 hours, or on high for 3 1/2. Blend and serve topped with fresh parsley.

## Cheesy Cauliflower Soup

**Serves 4**

**Prep time: 1 min**

**Cooking time: 5-6 hours**

**Ingredients:**

1 onion, chopped

1 head cauliflower, cut in florets

2 garlic cloves, minced

3 cups water

1 cup whole cream

1 cup cheddar cheese, grated

a pinch of thyme

salt, to taste

black pepper, to taste

**Directions:**

Put cauliflower, onion, garlic and water in the slow cooker. Cover and cook on low for 5-6 hours.

Blend in a blender, return to crockpot and stir in cream and cheese. Season with salt and pepper, stir to mix, and serve.

## Mediterranean Lentil Soup

**Serves: 4-5**

**Prep time: 35 min**

**Ingredients:**

1 cup red lentils

2 carrots, chopped

1 onion, chopped

1 garlic clove, chopped

1 small red pepper, chopped

3 ripe tomatoes, diced

½ can chickpeas, drained and rinsed (Note: Opt for BPA-free cans)

½ can white beans, drained and rinsed (Note: Opt for BPA-free cans)

1 small celery stalk, chopped

6 cups water

1 tbsp paprika

1 tsp ginger, grated

1 tsp cumin

3 tbsp extra virgin olive oil

**Directions:**

Heat olive oil in a deep soup pot and gently sauté onions, garlic, red pepper and ginger. Add in water, lentils, chickpeas, white beans, tomatoes, carrots, celery, and cumin.

Bring to a boil then lower heat and simmer for 35 minutes, or until the lentils are tender. Purée half the soup in a food processor. Return the puréed soup to the pot, stir and serve.

## Bean and Pasta Soup

**Serves: 4-5**

**Prep time: 10-15 min**

**Ingredients:**

1 onion, chopped

2 large carrots, chopped

2 garlic cloves, minced

1 cup cooked orzo

1 15 oz can white beans, rinsed and drained (Note: Opt for BPA-free cans)

3 ripe tomatoes, diced

1 cup baby spinach leaves

3 cups water

1 tbsp paprika

1 tbsp dried mint

3 tbsp extra virgin olive oil

salt and black pepper, to taste

**Directions:**

Heat the olive oil over medium heat and gently sauté the onion, garlic and carrots. Add in tomatoes, water, salt and pepper, and bring to a boil. Reduce heat and cook for 5-10 minutes, or until the carrots are tender. Stir in orzo, beans and spinach, and simmer until the spinach is wilted.

## Tuscan-style Bean Soup

**Serves: 4-5**

**Prep time: 10-15 min**

**Ingredients:**

1 onion, chopped

1 large carrot, chopped

2 garlic cloves, minced

1 15 oz can white beans, rinsed and drained (Note: Opt for BPA-free cans)

1 cup spinach leaves, trimmed and washed

3 cups water

1 tbsp paprika

1 tbsp dried mint

3 tbsp extra virgin olive oil

salt and black pepper, to taste

**Directions:**

Heat the olive oil over medium heat and gently sauté the onion, garlic and carrot. Add in beans, water, salt and pepper and bring to a boil.

Reduce heat and cook for 10 minutes, or until the carrots are tender. Stir in spinach, and simmer for about 5 minutes, until the spinach is wilted.

## Italian Vegetable Soup

**Serves: 4-5**

**Prep time: 25 min**

**Ingredients:**

1/2 onion, chopped

2 garlic cloves, chopped

¼ cabbage, chopped

1 carrot, chopped

2 celery stalks, chopped

4 cups water

3 ripe tomatoes, diced

1 1/2 cup green beans, trimmed and cut into 1/2-inch pieces

1/2 cup small pasta, cooked

2-3 fresh basil leaves

2 tbsp extra virgin olive oil

black pepper and salt, to taste

**Directions:**

Heat the olive oil in a large pot over medium-high heat. Add the onion and cook until translucent, about 4 minutes. Add in garlic, carrot and celery and cook for 5 minutes more.

Stir in the green beans, cabbage, tomatoes, basil, and water and bring to a boil. Reduce heat and simmer uncovered, for 15 minutes, or until the vegetables are tender.

Stir in pasta, season with pepper and salt to taste and serve.

## French Vegetable Soup

**Serves: 4-5**

**Prep time: 25 min**

**Ingredients:**

2 leeks, white and pale green parts only, well rinsed and thinly sliced

1 large zucchini, peeled and diced

1 medium fennel bulb, trimmed, cored, and cut into large chunks

2 garlic cloves, chopped

3 cups water

2 tomatoes, diced

1/2 cup vermicelli, broken into small pieces

3 tbsp extra virgin olive oil

black pepper, to taste

**Directions:**

Heat the olive oil in a large stockpot. Add the leeks and sauté over low heat for 5 minutes. Add in the zucchini, fennel and garlic and cook for about 5 minutes.

Stir in water and the tomatoes and bring to the boil. Reduce heat and simmer, uncovered, for 20 minutes, or until the vegetables are tender but still holding their shape. Stir in the vermicelli. Simmer for a further 5 minutes and serve.

## Spiced Beet and Carrot Soup

**Serves: 4-5**

**Prep time: 25 min**

**Ingredients:**

3 beets, washed and peeled

2 carrots, peeled and chopped

1 small onion, chopped

1 garlic clove, chopped

4 cups water

2 tbsp extra virgin olive oil

1 tsp grated ginger

1 tsp grated orange peel

**Directions:**

Heat the olive oil in a large stockpot. Add the onion and sauté over low heat for 3-4 minutes or until translucent. Add in garlic, beets, carrots, ginger, lemon rind and water and bring to the boil.

Reduce heat to medium and simmer, partially covered, for 30 minutes, or until the beets are tender. Cool slightly and blend soup in batches until smooth. Season with salt and pepper and serve.

## Clean Eating Main Dish Recipes

## Walnut Pesto Stuffed Chicken

**Serves: 4**

**Prep time: 35 min**

**Ingredients:**

4 large chicken breasts

**for the walnut pesto**

1/2 cup walnuts, chopped

10 fresh basil leaves

1 garlic clove

2-3 green olives

4 tbsp extra virgin olive oil

1 tbsp lemon juice

salt and black pepper, to taste

**Directions:**

In a food processor, blend together walnuts, olives, basil, olive oil, garlic and lemon juice until completely smooth.

Carefully butterfly each chicken breast. Cover with plastic wrap and beat with a heavy object until the breast is flattened.

Put a tablespoon of the walnut mixture in each breast and roll over the top part like a flap. Season with salt and black pepper and bake at 375 F for 35 minutes.

## Chicken with Olive Paste

**Serves: 4**

**Prep time: 40 min**

**Ingredients:**

2 chicken breasts (each cut into 2 cutlets)

2 garlic cloves, crushed

**for the olive paste:**

2 tbsp olive oil

2 cloves garlic, peeled

2/3 cup pitted black olives

2 tbsp capers

1 tbsp tomato paste

1 tbsp basil, chopped

3 tbsp extra virgin olive oil

salt and pepper, to taste

**Directions:**

Place the garlic cloves into a food processor together with the olives, capers, basil, tomato paste and olive oil. Blend until smooth. Season to taste with salt and pepper.

Gently heat oil in a skillet on medium heat. Add in the chicken cutlets and cook each side for 4-5 minutes. Serve each cutlet topped with olive paste.

## Chicken and Chickpea Casserole

**Serves: 4**

**Prep time: 40 min**

*Ingredients*:

8 chicken drumsticks

2 leeks, trimmed, thinly sliced

1 garlic clove, crushed

1 can chickpeas, drained and rinsed (Note: Opt for BPA-free cans)

3 ripe tomatoes, diced

1 tsp dried rosemary

3 tbsp extra virgin olive oil

cooked couscous, to serve

**Directions:**

In a casserole, gently heat the oil over medium-high heat. Brown the chicken tights for 1-2 minutes, each side.

Add in leeks and garlic and cook, stirring, for 2 minutes or until soft. Add in the tomatoes, chickpeas, and rosemary and bring to a boil.

Cover and simmer for 35 minutes or until the chicken is tender. Season with salt and pepper and serve with couscous.

## Greek Chicken Casserole

**Serves: 4**

**Prep time: 45 min**

**Ingredients:**

8 chicken tights

1 onion, chopped

4-5 potatoes, peeled and cubed

1 carrot, chopped

1 lb green beans, trimmed and chopped

1 cup diced, tomatoes

2 garlic cloves, chopped

1 cup feta cheese, crumbled

3 tbsp extra virgin olive oil

salt and black pepper, to taste

**Directions:**

Heat oil in a large casserole dish over medium heat. Add in onion and chicken and cook for a minute, stirring. Add in black pepper, carrot and garlic and sauté for another minute. Add potatoes and cook for 2 minutes, or until they begin to brown. Stir in beans and tomatoes.

Sprinkle with salt and black pepper to taste and top with feta. Cover, and bake for 40 minutes, stirring halfway through.

## Chicken Puttanesca

**Serves: 4**

**Prep time: 30 min**

**Ingredients:**

4 boneless chicken breasts

2 tbsp extra virgin olive oil

**for the sauce:**

2 tbsp extra virgin olive oil

4 garlic cloves, crushed

1 small onion, diced

1/2 cup green olives, pitted and chopped

2 tbsp capers, drained and coarsely chopped

3 boneless anchovy fillets, coarsely chopped

2 tomatoes, diced

1 tbsp tomato paste

1 tbsp paprika

salt and black pepper, to taste

**Directions:**

Heat two tablespoons of olive oil in a large skillet and brown the chicken for about 2 minutes, each side. Cover with a lid and cook for about 10-15 minutes, or until cooked through. Set aside on 4 plates.

In the same skillet, heat two tablespoons of olive oil. Add in garlic, onions, anchovies, olives, capers and paprika. Gently sauté these ingredients, stirring constantly, for about one minute. Add in the tomatoes and tomato paste, season with salt and pepper and cook over high heat for 5-6 minutes or until the tomatoes are cooked and the sauce thickens. Divide the sauce between the chicken breasts and serve.

## Meatballs with Tomato Sauce

**Serves: 4-5**

**Prep time: 30 min**

**Ingredients:**

2 lbs ground beef

1 onion,very finely cut

2 eggs, lightly whisked

1 tbsp chia seeds

1 tbsp parsley, finely chopped

1/2 tsp cumin

1/2 tsp ground ginger

4 ripe tomatoes, diced

2 tbsp tomato paste

1 cup water

2 tbsp extra virgin olive oil

salt, to taste

**Directions:**

Preheat the oven to 350 F. Line a baking tray with baking paper.

Combine the ground beef, onion, eggs, chia seeds, parsley, salt and cumin in a bowl. Using your hands, mix everything until it well combined. Roll beef mixture into walnut sized meatballs and arrange them on the baking tray. Bake for 10 minutes until light golden.

In a deep saucepan, heat olive oil over medium heat. Stir in ginger, tomatoes and tomato paste. Add water and bring to a boil, then reduce heat and simmer for 5 minutes. Add the meatballs and simmer for 20 more minutes or until the meat is cooked through and the sauce has thickened.

## Mediterranean Meatloaf with Vegetables

**Serves: 4-5**

**Prep time: 45 min**

**Ingredients:**

2 lbs ground beef

2 eggs, lightly beaten

1/3 cup almond meal

1 zucchini, peeled and diced

2 small tomatoes, halved

5-6 white mushrooms, halved

2 small onions, peeled and quartered

2-3 small parsnips

1/3 cup homemade chicken broth

4 tbsp extra virgin olive oil

1 cup fresh parsley, finely cut

1 tsp dried oregano

1 tsp garlic powder

salt and black pepper, to taste

**Directions:**

Place ground beef, eggs, almond meal, parsley, salt, garlic powder and black pepper in a bowl and combine well with hands. Prepare a loaf and place it in the center of a baking dish.

Arrange vegetables around the meatloaf, add in chicken broth, sprinkle with dried oregano and season with salt to taste. Bake in a preheated to 350 F oven for 40 minutes.

## Ground Beef and Brussels Sprouts

**Serves: 4**

**Prep time: 20 min**

**Ingredients:**

6 oz ground beef

1/2 onion, finely cut

2 garlic cloves, crushed

½ cup grated sweet potato

1 cup grated Brussels sprouts

1 egg, boiled

1 tbsp extra virgin olive oil

**Directions:**

In a medium saucepan, heat the olive oil over medium heat. Gently sauté the onion and garlic until the onion is soft and translucent. Add in the beef and the sweet potato and cook until the meat is fully cooked.

Stir in the Brussels sprouts and cook for about 5 minutes more. Season with salt and pepper to taste and serve topped with a boiled egg.

## Hearty Meatball Stew

**Serves: 6**

**Prep time: 35 min**

**Ingredients:**

**for the meatballs:**

2 lbs ground beef

1 onion, finely copped

1/3 cup parsley leaves, finely chopped

**for the sauce:**

1/2 small onion, chopped

1 carrot, chopped

1 red pepper, cut

1 zucchini, peeled and cut

1/2 eggplant, peeled and diced

2 garlic cloves, chopped

4 white mushrooms, sliced

4 ripe tomatoes, diced

1/2 cup water

tbsp extra virgin olive oil

1/2 cup parsley leaves, to serve

salt and black pepper, to taste

**Directions:**

Combine ground beef, onion, parsley, salt and pepper in a bowl. Roll tablespoonfuls of beef mixture into balls and set aside on plate.

Heat olive oil in a saucepan. Gently sauté the onion, pepper, carrot and garlic for 2-3 minutes, stirring. Add in the mushrooms, eggplant and zucchini, stir and cook for 2-3 minutes more. Add in tomatoes and water and bring to a boil over medium heat.

Drop beef meatballs into the tomato mixture. Reduce heat to low and simmer, uncovered, for 30 minutes or until the meatballs are cooked through. Sprinkle with parsley and serve.

## Italian Mini Meatballs

**Serves: 6**

**Prep time: 35 min**

**Ingredients:**

1 lb ground beef

1 onion, grated

1 egg, lightly whisked

1 tbsp dried parsley

1 tsp garlic powder

1 tsp dried basil

1 tsp dried oregano

1/4 cup olive oil

**Directions:**

Combine ground beef, onion, egg, parsley, garlic powder, basil and oregano. Mix very well with hands. Roll tablespoonfuls of the meat mixture into balls.

Place meatballs on a lined baking tray. Bake 20 minutes or until brown. Transfer to a serving plate and serve with vegetable salad.

## Mediterranean Steak

**Serves 4**

**Prep time: 20 min**

**Ingredients:**

4 sirloin steaks, trimmed

6 large tomatoes, sliced

1 onion, sliced

2 tsp baby capers

1 tbsp dried basil

3 garlic cloves, crushed

1 tbsp lemon juice

1/4 cup extra virgin olive oil

salt and black pepper, to taste

**Directions:**

Place steaks in a shallow dish. Rub both sides with half the olive oil, garlic, herbs, and black pepper. Set aside in a refrigerator for 1 hour.

Preheat oven to 350 F. Arrange tomatoes on a baking tray lined with baking paper. Scatter over capers and onion slices. Sprinkle with the remaining olive oil and cook for 15 minutes.

Heat a non-stick grill pan over high heat. Cook steaks to desired doneness, 4 minutes per side for rare.

Serve on a bed of roasted tomatoes and onions.

## Italian Pot Roast

**Serves 6**

**Prep time: 120 min**

**Ingredients:**

4 garlic cloves, crushed

2 onions, sliced

6 carrots, quartered

4 celery ribs, cut into thick pieces

2 bay leaves

1 tbsp finely chopped rosemary

1/4 tsp black pepper

1 tbsp dried basil

1 tbsp dried oregano

1/4 cup olive oil

**Directions:**

Combine all the spice in a small bowl. Heat the olive oil in a large oven-proof dish and immediately seal all sides of the roast. Coat it with the spice mix.

Put roast in the middle of the baking dish. Crush the garlic and add it to the dish together with the onions, bay leaves, carrots and celery.

Cover and bake at 325 degrees 1 1/2 -2 hours, or until cooked to your liking.

## Roast Beef with Quince, Parsnips and Carrots

**Serves 6**

**Prep time: 60-70 min**

**Ingredients:**

2-3 lb roast beef round

4 parsnips, peeled, quartered lengthwise

6 carrots, quartered lengthwise

2 quinces, peeled, cored and cubed

1 cup homemade beef or chicken broth

2 tbsp apple puree

1 tbsp Dijon mustard

3 tbsp extra virgin olive oil

black pepper, to taste

**Directions:**

Whisk together beef broth, apple puree and mustard until smooth.

Heat the olive oil in a large frying pan over high heat and seal all sides of the roast.

Transfer roast to a baking dish.

Arrange the parsnips around the beef. Sprinkle with black pepper and roast for 15 minutes. Add in the carrots and roast, stirring the vegetables once, for a further 25 minutes. Add in the quince. Brush the beef with the apple puree and mustard mixture.

Cover and bake at 325 degrees 30 minutes, or until cooked to your liking.

## Eggplant With Ground Beef

**Serves: 6**

**Prep time: 45 min**

**Ingredients:**

1 lb ground beef

2 eggplants, peeled and cut into thick rounds

1 tbsp salt

1 onion, chopped

2 garlic cloves, crushed

1/2 tsp ground cinnamon

1/2 tsp ground nutmeg

1/4 tsp ground coriander

2 ripe tomatoes, diced

1/2 cup parsley leaves, finely chopped

2 eggs

3 tbsp milk

4 tbsp extra virgin olive oil

salt and black pepper, to taste

**Directions:**

Peel and cut the eggplant and place the slices on a plate. Sprinkle with a tablespoon of salt and set aside for 30 minutes, then rinse and pat dry.

Heat olive oil in a deep frying pan over medium-high heat. Fry the eggplant slices in batches for 2-3 minutes each side or until golden. Set aside in a plate.

In the same pan, sauté onion and garlic for 2-3 minutes or until transparent. Add in ground beef and spice, mix well and sauté until it turns light brown. Add in tomatoes and parsley and simmer until the sauce thickens.

Place half the eggplant slices in an ovenproof baking dish. Cover with beef and tomato mixture and top with remaining eggplant.

Whisk two eggs with milk. Pour over the meat and eggplant mixture. Bake for 30 minutes or until golden. Set aside for five minutes and serve.

## Steak with Olives and Mushrooms

**Serves: 6**

**Prep time: 20 min**

**Ingredients:**

1 lb boneless beef sirloin steak, 3/4-inch thick, cut into 4 pieces

1 large onion, sliced

5-6 white mushrooms

1/2 cup green olives, coarsely chopped

4 tbsp extra virgin olive oil

1 cup parsley leaves, finely cut

**Directions:**

Heat olive oil in a heavy bottomed skillet over medium-high heat. Cook the steaks until well browned on both sides then set aside in a plate.

Gently sauté the onion in the same skillet, for 2-3 minutes, stirring occasionally. Add in the mushrooms and olives and cook until the mushrooms are done.

Return the steaks to the skillet, cover, and cook for 5-6 minutes. Stir in parsley and serve.

## Mediterranean Beef Casserole

**Serves: 5-6**

**Prep time: 80 min**

**Ingredients:**

2 lbs boneless lean beef stew meat, cut into 1 1/2-inch cubes

1 onion, sliced

2 garlic cloves, chopped

2 carrots, cut

1 fennel bulb, trimmed and thinly sliced vertically

1 zucchini, cut

3 tomatoes, quartered

2 tbsp tomato paste

1/2 cup black olives, pitted

1/2 cup water

2 tbsp extra virgin olive oil

1 bay leaf

1 tsp dried basil

salt and black pepper, to taste

**Directions:**

Heat the olive oil in a deep saucepan and brown the beef. Dilute the tomato paste in the water and pour over the beef mixture.

Add in the olives, bay leaf and basil and simmer, covered, for 60 minutes. Add all vegetables and simmer for 20 minutes more.

## Herb-Roasted Lamb Leg

**Serves 4**

**Prep time: 130 min**

**Ingredients:**

1 (6-lb) boneless leg of lamb, trimmed

2 cups fresh spinach leaves

4-5 garlic cloves, crushed

1 bay leaf

1 cup fresh mint

1/2 tsp thyme

1 tsp fresh rosemary leaves

1/3 cup water

1 tsp black pepper

1 tsp salt

4 tbsp extra virgin olive oil

**Directions:**

Combine garlic, spinach, herbs, salt, black pepper and olive oil in a food processor. Process until finely minced.

Thoroughly coat the top and sides of the lamb with this mixture.

Place in the bottom of a large roasting pan. Add water and cook, covered, at 300 F for approximately two hours or until cooked through.

Uncover and cook for 10 minutes more.

## Lamb Asparagus Stew

**Serves 4**

**Prep time: 30-40 min**

**Ingredients:**

1 lb cubed lamb

2 lbs fresh asparagus, trimmed and cut into 2 inch pieces

1 lb shallots

1 cup water

juice of 1 lemon

1 tsp dry mint

1 tsp dry oregano

salt and black pepper, to taste

3 tbsp extra virgin olive oil

**Directions:**

Wash and trim asparagus. Cut into 2 inch pieces.

Heat olive oil in a deep casserole and brown lamb pieces on moderate heat. Add in shallots and cook for a few minutes.

Add water and herbs, cover, and cook for an hour or until the meat is tender.

Stir in asparagus. Season with salt and black pepper to taste and cook for 6-7 minutes more. Add lemon juice and serve.

## Spring Lamb Stew

**Serves 4**

**Prep time: 30-40 min**

**Ingredients:**

1 lb lamb, cubed

1 lb white mushrooms, chopped

4 cups fresh spring onions, chopped

1 tomato, chopped

3 tbsp extra virgin olive oil

1 tbsp paprika

1 cup fresh mint, finely cut

3 cups fresh parsley, finely cut

**Directions:**

Heat olive oil in a deep casserole. Gently brown lamb pieces for 2-3 minutes. Add in mushrooms and cook for a minute more, stirring.

Stir in paprika, cover, and cook for an hour or until tender. Add in spring onions, tomatoes, mint and parsley and simmer for 10 minutes more.

Uncover and cook until almost all the liquid evaporates.

## Lamb Tagine with Green Olives and Lemon

**Serves 4**

**Prep time: 30-40 min**

**Ingredients:**

3 lb boneless lamb shoulder, cut into 1-inch pieces

4-5 large carrots, thinly sliced

1 onion, chopped

2 garlic cloves, crushed

2 cups green olives, pitted

3 cups water

3 tbsp extra virgin olive oil

1 tbsp lemon zest

1 tbsp paprika

1 tsp cumin

1 tsp ground coriander

1 tsp cinnamon

a pinch of saffron threads, crumbled

1 tsp black pepper

1 tsp salt

3 tbsp lemon juice

1 cup cilantro leaves, chopped

1/2 cup fresh mint, finely cut

**Directions:**

coriander, cumin, black pepper, saffron, cinnamon and salt. Add the lamb and toss to coat. Refrigerate for at least 4 hours.

Place the lamb and spices into a tagine or a casserole. Add the water, carrots and onion and bring to a boil. Cover and simmer over low heat until the lamb is tender, about 2 hours.

Stir in the olives and cook for 2 minutes. Stir in the mint, cilantro and lemon juice and serve.

## Beef Tagine with Sweet Potatoes

**Serves: 4-5**

**Prep time: 120 min**

**Ingredients:**

2 lbs stewing beef

1 onion, finely chopped

1/2 cup water

1 bunch of fresh cilantro

1 bunch of fresh parsley

2 ripe tomatoes, peeled and sliced

1 lb sweet potatoes, peeled and cut into slices

4-5 tbsp extra virgin olive oil

½ tsp turmeric

½ tsp black pepper

1/2 tsp paprika

1/4 tsp ground ginger

½ tsp cumin

**Directions:**

In an deep casserole dish, heat olive oil and sauté the beef until well browned. Add in onion, water, turmeric, salt, black pepper and all remaining spices.

Tie the parsley and cilantro together into a bouquet and place on top of the beef. Cover, bring to a boil, immediately reduce heat, and simmer for 60 minutes until the meat is tender.

add the sweet potatoes on top of the beef. Place the tomatoes on top of the sweet potatoes. Cover again and simmer for 40 minutes, until the meat and potatoes are tender.

## Slow Cooked Beef Couscous

**Serves 5-6**

**Prep time: 2 min**

**Cooking time: 7-9 hours**

**Ingredients:**

2 lbs stewing beef

1 onion, cut

1/2 cup canned chickpeas, drained (Note: Opt for BPA-free cans)

2 carrots, cut

1/2 cup green peas

1/2 cup black olives, pitted

3 tbsp tomato paste

2 cups water

1 zucchini, peeled and cut

1 cup frozen green beans

3 potatoes, peeled and cut

1 tsp cumin

1 tsp paprika

a small bunch of fresh parsley

**Directions:**

Place beef, onion, chickpeas, green peas, carrot, olives, tomato paste, cumin, paprika and water in slow cooker. Tie the parsley into a bouquet and place it on top. Cover and cook on low for 10 hours.

pepper to taste, increase heat setting to high and cook for 1 hour more. In the end discard the parsley bouquet.

Serve over cooked couscous with meat and vegetables on top and stew sauce in a separate bowl.

## Easy Beef Crock Pot

**Serves 4**

**Prep time: 2 min**

**Cooking time: 7-9 hours**

**Ingredients:**

2 lbs beef, cubed

3 leeks, finely cut

1 celery rib, finely cut

10 white button mushrooms, sliced

1 cup milk

1 tsp dried thyme

1 tsp salt

1/2 tsp black pepper

2 tbsp extra virgin olive oil

**Directions:**

Spray the slow cooker with non stick spray.

In a skillet, brown the beef for 1-2 minutes or until sealed.

Combine all ingredients into the slow cooker, cover, and cook on low for 7-9 hours.

## Stuffed Bell Peppers

**Serves: 4-5**

**Prep time: 40 min**

**Ingredients:**

1 lb lean ground beef

5-6 red bell peppers

1 onion, grated

2 garlic cloves, chopped

1 tomato, diced

1/3 cup pine nuts, toasted

5 tbsp extra virgin olive oil

1/2 cup finely cut parsley

1/3 cup water

1 tbsp paprika

salt and pepper, to taste

**Directions:**

Heat olive oil in a skillet pot and gently sauté onions and garlic until transparent. Add in ground beef, paprika, tomato, parsley, and pine nuts. Cook for 2-3 minutes, stirring. Season with salt and pepper and remove from heat.

Spoon beef mixture into peppers. Arrange the stuffed peppers in a deep pot in one layer. Add in water and bing to a boil. Reduce heat and simmer for about 30 minutes.

## Ground Beef and Cabbage Casserole

**Serves: 4-5**

**Prep time: 50 min**

**Ingredients:**

1 lb ground beef

1/2 cabbage, shredded

1/2 onion, chopped

2 leeks, white part only, chopped

1 tomato, diced

1 tbsp paprika

1/2 tsp cumin

½ tsp black pepper

4 tbsp extra virgin olive oil

salt, to taste

**Directions:**

In a deep saucepan, sauté the onion and leeks in olive oil until tender. Add in the ground beef, tomato, paprika, cumin, salt and black pepper.

Place the shredded cabbage on the bottom of an ovenproof baking dish. Cover with beef mixture. Cover with a lid or aluminum foil and bake at 325 F for 40 minutes.

## Ground Beef and Lentil Casserole

**Serves: 4-5**

**Prep time: 30 min**

**Ingredients:**

1 lb ground beef

1 small onion, chopped

2 garlic cloves, crushed

1 cup dry green lentils

1 carrot, chopped

2 cups water

2 bay leaves

1 tsp dried oregano

1 tbsp paprika

1/2 tsp salt

1/2 tsp cumin

3 tbsp extra virgin olive oil

black pepper, to taste

**Directions:**

Heat the olive oil in a casserole over medium-high heat. Add the onion and carrot and sauté for 4-5 minutes. Add in garlic and sauté a minute more. Add the ground beef and cook for 4-5 minutes, stirring, until browned. Add the paprika, cumin, oregano, bay leaves, tomatoes, lentils and water.

Bring everything to a boil then reduce heat and simmer for 20 minutes, or until the beef is cooked through. Remove the bay leaves and serve.

## Salmon Kebabs

**Serves: 4-5**

**Prep time: 30 min**

**Ingredients:**

2 shallots, ends trimmed, halved

2 zucchinis, cut in 2 inch cubes

1 cup cherry tomatoes

6 skinless salmon fillets, cut into 1 inch pieces

3 limes, cut into thin wedges

**Directions:**

Preheat barbecue or char grill on medium-high. Thread fish cubes onto skewers, then zucchinis, shallots and tomatoes. Repeat to make 12 kebabs. Bake the kebabs for about 3 minutes each side for medium cooked.

Transfer to a plate, cover with foil and set aside for 5 minutes to rest.

## Salmon and Spinach with Feta Cheese

**Serves: 4**

**Prep time: 15 min**

**Ingredients:**

4 salmon fillets, skin on

1 bag frozen spinach

4-5 green onions, chopped

1 cup crumbled feta cheese

4 tbsp extra virgin olive oil

salt and pepper, to taste

lemon wedges, to serve

**Directions:**

In a skillet, heat olive oil on medium-high. Cook the spinach and the green onions for 2-3 min, stirring once or twice. Season with salt and pepper to taste and add in the feta cheese. Cook for 1 minute more.

Place salmon skin side down in a single layer on a lined baking tray and roast for 10-12 minutes or until it is cooked through and flakes easily with a fork.

Spoon the spinach mixture onto plates, then top with the salmon and serve with lemon wedges.

## Almond and Oregano Crusted Fish Fillets

**Serves: 4**

**Prep time: 10 min**

**Ingredients:**

4 white fish fillets

1 tsp dried oregano

1/2 cup raw almonds, chopped

1 garlic clove, chopped

2 tbsp grated Parmesan cheese

3 egg whites, beaten

salt and pepper, to taste

**Directions:**

Blend the garlic, Parmesan cheese, oregano and almonds in a food processor until a light crumb is formed. Stir in salt and black pepper and place on a plate.

Whisk egg whites in a deep bowl. Dip each fish fillet in the beaten egg whites then roll it in the almond mixture.

Place coated fish on a lined baking tray and bake at 375 F for 6-7 minutes each side.

## Feta Cheese Baked in Foil

**Serves: 4**

**Prep time: 15 min**

**Ingredients:**

14 oz feta cheese, cut in slices

4 oz butter

1 tbsp paprika

1 tsp dried oregano

aluminum foil, enough to cover 4 slices of cheese

**Directions:**

Cut the cheese into four medium-thick slices and place on sheets of butter lined aluminum foil.

Place a little bit of butter on top each feta cheese piece, sprinkle with paprika and dried oregano and wrap. Place on a tray and bake in a preheated to 350 F oven for 15 minutes.

## Spicy Baked Feta with Tomatoes

**Serves: 4**

**Prep time: 15 min**

**Ingredients:**

1 lb feta cheese, cut in slices

2 ripe tomatoes, sliced

1 red pepper, sliced

1 onion, sliced

3 tbsp extra virgin olive oil

1/2 tbsp hot paprika

1 tsp dried oregano

**Directions:**

Preheat the oven to 430F

In an ovenproof baking dish, arrange the slices of onions, tomatoes, and pepper overlapping slightly but not too much. Sprinkle with olive oil, salt and black pepper to taste.

Bake for 5 minutes then place the feta slices on top of the vegetables. Sprinkle with oregano and hot paprika. Bake for 15 more minutes and serve.

## Creamy Avocado Spaghetti

**Serves: 5-6**

**Prep time: 20 min**

**Ingredients:**

12 oz spaghetti

1/2 cup black olives, halved

1 red pepper, cut in thin strips

2 avocados, peeled and diced

1 cup cherry tomatoes, halved

2 cloves garlic, finely chopped

1 tbsp basil pesto

5 tbsp extra virgin olive oil

4 tbsp lemon juice

1/4 cup grated Parmesan cheese

**Directions:**

In a large pot of boiling salted water, cook spaghetti according to package instructions. Drain and set aside in a large bowl.

In a blender, combine lemon juice, garlic, basil pesto and avocados and blend until smooth.

Combine spaghetti, olives, cherry tomatoes, red pepper, and avocado sauce. Sprinkle with Parmesan cheese and serve immediately.

## Tomato, Arugula and Feta Spaghetti

**Serves: 5-6**

**Prep time: 20 min**

**Ingredients:**

12 oz spaghetti

2 cups grape tomatoes, halved

1 cup fresh basil leaves, roughly torn

1 cup baby arugula leaves

1 cup feta, crumbled

2 garlic cloves, chopped

5 tbsp extra virgin olive oil

salt and black pepper, to taste

**Directions:**

In a large saucepan of boiling salted water, cook spaghetti according to package instructions. Drain and set aside in a large bowl.

Return saucepan to medium heat. Add olive oil, garlic and tomatoes. Season with pepper and cook, tossing, for 1-2 minutes or until tomatoes are hot. Add spaghetti, basil and feta. Toss gently for 1 minute or until heated through. Sprinkle with arugula and serve.

## Mediterranean Pizza

**Serves: 4**

**Prep time: 35 min**

**Ingredients:**

1 store-bought or homemade dough

3-4 green onions, chopped

1 (6 oz) can quartered artichoke hearts, drained and rinsed (Note: Opt for BPA-free cans)

1/2 cup red bell pepper, chopped

1 garlic clove, chopped

1 cup black olives, chopped

1 cup baby arugula leaves

1/2 cup fresh tomato sauce

1 cup (4 oz) crumbled goat or Parmesan cheese

3 tbsp extra virgin olive oil

1 tbsp dried basil

salt and black pepper, to taste

**Directions:**

Heat a large skillet on medium heat and sauté the onion and bell pepper for 2-3 minutes until fragrant. Add in the artichoke hearts, garlic, olives and basil and sauté for 5 minutes more. Season with salt and black pepper to taste.

Roll out dough onto a floured surface and transfer to a parchment-lined 12 inch round baking sheet.

Top it with tomato sauce, goat cheese and the sautéed vegetables.

Bake for 30 minutes in a preheated to 450 F oven or until the crust is golden brown and the sauce is bubbly. Set aside for 5 minutes, cut, and serve.

## Delicious Zucchini Pasta

**Serves: 4-5**

**Prep time: 35 min**

**Ingredients:**

12 oz dry pasta

1 small onion, chopped

2 zucchinis, peeled and cubed

2-3 garlic cloves, crushed

1.5 cups marinara sauce

1 cup black olives, pitted

2 tbsp capers

2 cups water

3 tbsp extra virgin olive oil

1 cup grated Parmesan cheese

1/2 cup fresh dill, finely cut

1 tsp salt

1 tsp fresh black pepper

**Directions:**

Heat a deep saucepan over medium-high heat. Add in olive oil and gently sauté the onion, garlic and zucchinis. Stir in water, marinara sauce and pasta.

Season with salt and black pepper, bring to a boil, cover, and simmer until the pasta is cooked to al dente. Sprinkle with fresh dill, capers, Parmesan cheese, and serve.

## Easy One-Pot Spaghetti

**Serves: 4-5**

**Ingredients:**

12 oz spaghetti

1/2 onion, chopped

1 lb boneless chicken breast half, cooked and diced

1 (6 oz) can artichoke hearts, drained and rinsed (Note: Opt for BPA-free cans)

1/2 can chickpeas, drained

2 garlic cloves, crushed

1.5 cups tomato sauce

2 cups water

3 tbsp extra virgin olive oil

1 tsp dried basil

1 tsp dried oregano

1/3 cup fresh parsley, finely cut

1/3 cup crumbled feta cheese

**Directions:**

Heat a large saucepan over medium-high heat. Add in olive oil and gently sauté the onion, garlic, chicken, chickpeas, artichoke hearts, water, and tomato sauce. Season with salt and black pepper and bring to a boil.

Add in spaghetti, basil and oregano, and stir. Reduce heat and simmer until the spaghetti is cooked to al dente.

Sprinkle with parsley and feta cheese, and serve.

## Hearty Lentil Spaghetti

**Serves: 4-5**

**Prep time: 35 min**

**Ingredients:**

12 oz spaghetti

1/2 onion, chopped

1 can brown lentils, rinsed and drained (Note: Opt for BPA-free cans)

1 cup green olives, pitted and halved

1-2 garlic cloves, chopped

2 cups tomato sauce

2 cups water

3 tbsp extra virgin olive oil

1/3 cup fresh mint, finely cut

1 tsp salt

1 cup crumbled feta cheese

**Directions:**

Heat a deep saucepan over medium-high heat. Add in olive oil and gently sauté the onion, garlic, lentils, olives, water and tomato sauce.

Bring to a boil, then add spaghetti and stir. Reduce heat and simmer until the spaghetti is cooked to al dente.

Sprinkle with feta cheese and mint, adjust seasonings, and serve.

## Spicy Chickpea and Spinach Stew

**Serves: 4**

**Prep time: 40 min**

**Ingredients:**

1 onion, chopped

3 garlic cloves, chopped

1 15 oz can chickpeas, drained and rinsed (Note: Opt for BPA-free cans)

3 ripe tomatoes, diced

1 1 lb bag baby spinach

a handful of blanched almonds

½ cup water

1 tbsp tomato paste

1 tbsp hot chilli paste

½ tsp cumin

salt and pepper, to taste

**Directions:**

Heat olive oil in a large saucepan over medium-high heat. Gently sauté onion and garlic for 4-5 minutes, or until tender. Add spices and stir. Add in chickpeas, tomatoes, almonds and the tomato paste dissolved in the water.

Bring to a boil, then reduce heat to low and simmer, partially covered, for 10 minutes. Add the chilli paste and spinach to the pot and stir until the spinach wilts. Remove from heat and season with salt and pepper to taste.

## Moroccan Chickpea Stew

**Serves: 4-5**

**Prep time: 20 min**

**Ingredients:**

1 onion, chopped

3 garlic cloves, chopped

2 large carrots, chopped

2 potatoes, peeled and chopped

4-5 dates, pitted and chopped

1 cup spinach, chopped

3 ripe tomatoes, diced

1 15 oz can chickpeas, rinsed and drained, (Note: Opt for BPA-free cans)

1 cup water

1 tbsp ground cumin

½ tsp chilli powder

½ tsp ground turmeric

½ teaspoon salt

3 tbsp extra virgin olive oil

½ cup chopped cilantro, to serve

grated lemon zest, to serve

**Directions:**

Heat olive oil in a large saucepan over medium-high heat. Gently sauté onion, garlic and carrots for 4-5 minutes, or until tender. Add all spices and stir. Stir in all other ingredients except the spinach. Bring to a boil, cover, reduce heat, and simmer for 20 minutes, or until potatoes are tender.

Add in spinach, stir and cook it until it wilts. Serve over brown rice, quinoa or couscous and top with chopped cilantro and lemon zest.

## Zucchini Fritters

**Serves: 4**

**Prep time: 20 min**

**Ingredients:**

5 zucchinis, grated

3 eggs

2 garlic cloves, crushed

5 spring onions, finely chopped

1 cup feta cheese, crumbled

1/2 cup fresh dill, finely cut

salt and black pepper, to taste

1 cup flour

1 cup sunflower oil

**Directions:**

Grate zucchinis and put them in a colander. Sprinkle with salt and leave aside to drain.

After 20 minutes, squeeze and place in a bowl. Add in all other ingredients except for the flour and sunflower oil. Combine everything very well. Add in flour and stir to combine again.

Heat the sunflower oil in a frying pan. Drop a few scoops of the zucchini batter and fry them on medium heat for 3-5 minutes, until golden brown. Serve with yogurt.

## Baked Falafels

**Serves: 7**

**Prep time: 20-30 min**

**Ingredients:**

1 can chickpeas, drained and rinsed (Note: Opt for BPA-free cans)

1 small carrot, cut

1 onion, cut

2 garlic cloves, minced

½ cup fresh parsley, finely cut

¼ cup whole wheat flour

¼ cup tahini

1/4 cup extra virgin olive oil

2-3 tbsp lemon juice

2 tsp cumin (or to taste)

1 tsp salt

black pepper, to taste

**Directions:**

Blend the carrots, chickpeas, onion and garlic in a food processor until completely minced. When it turns to a smooth paste, add in parsley and transfer to a large mixing bowl. Stir in the remaining ingredients.

Using a large tablespoon form batter into burgers. Bake in a preheated to 375F oven until golden.

## Chickpea, Rice and Mushroom Stew

**Serves: 4-5**

**Prep time: 20-30 min**

**Ingredients:**

1 15 oz can chickpeas, drained and rinsed, (Note: Opt for BPA-free cans)

1 large onion, finely cut

2 cups mushrooms, chopped

2 carrots, chopped

4 ripe tomatoes tomatoes, diced

1/3 cup rice, washed

1 cup water

4 tbsp extra virgin olive oil

1 tsp oregano

1 tbsp paprika

1 cup fresh parsley, finely cut

1 tbsp sugar

**Directions:**

In a deep, heavy-bottomed saucepan, heat olive oil and gently sauté the onion and carrots for 4-5 minutes, stirring constantly. Add in paprika, chickpeas, rice, mushrooms, tomatoes, sugar and water and stir again.

Season with salt, oregano, ground black pepper and bring to the boil. Cover, reduce heat, and simmer for about 20 minutes, stirring from time to time. Sprinkle with parsley, simmer for a minute more and serve.

## Balsamic Roasted Carrots and Baby Onions

**Serves: 4**

**Prep time: 50 min**

**Ingredients:**

2 bunches baby carrots, scrubbed, ends trimmed

10 small onions, peeled, halved

4 tbsp 100% pure maple syrup (unprocessed)

1 tsp thyme

2 tbsp extra virgin olive oil

**Directions:**

Preheat oven to 350F. Line a baking tray with baking paper.

Place the carrots, onion, thyme and oil in a large bowl and toss until well coated. Arrange carrots and onion, in a single layer, on the baking tray. Roast for 25 minutes or until tender.

Sprinkle over the maple syrup and vinegar and toss to coat. Roast for 25-30 minutes more or until vegetables are tender and caramelized. Season with salt and pepper to taste and serve.

## Ratatouille

**Serves: 4**

**Prep time: 45 min**

**Ingredients:**

1 eggplant, peeled and diced

2 large tomatoes, diced

2 zucchinis, peeled and sliced

1 onion, sliced

1 green pepper, sliced

6-7 mushrooms, sliced

3 cloves garlic, crushed

1 tbsp dried parsley

3 tbsp extra virgin olive oil

salt, to taste

**Directions:**

Place eggplant on a tray and sprinkle it with salt. Set aside for 30 minutes, then rinse and pat dry.

Heat olive oil in an ovenproof casserole dish over medium heat. Gently sauté garlic until fragrant.

Add in parsley and eggplant and cook until eggplant is soft. Spread zucchinis in an even layer over the eggplant. Layer onion, mushrooms, pepper and tomatoes, and bake in a preheated to 350 F oven for 40 minutes.

## Baked Bean and Rice Casserole

**Serves: 4-5**

**Prep time: 30 min**

**Ingredients:**

1 cup dried white or red beans, soaked in water overnight

1 cup water

2/3 cup rice

2 onions, chopped

1 cup parsley, finely cut

7-8 fresh mint leaves, finely cut

3 tbsp extra virgin olive oil

1 tbsp paprika

½ tsp black pepper

1 tsp salt

**Directions:**

Soak the beans in cold water overnight, drain and discard the water. Cover the beans with cold water again, bring to the boil and simmer until the beans are tender.

Heat olive oil in an ovenproof casserole dish and gently sauté the chopped onions for 1-2 minutes. Stir in paprika and rice and cook, stirring constantly, for another minute. Drain the beans and add them to the casserole.

Stir in and a cup of water, mint, parsley, season with salt and black pepper, and bake in a preheated to 350 F oven for 20 minutes.

## Baked Cauliflower

**Serves: 4**

**Prep time: 25 min**

**Ingredients:**

1 small cauliflower, cut into florets

1 tbsp garlic powder

1 tsp paprika

salt, to taste

black pepper, to taste

4 tbsp extra virgin olive oil

1/2 cup grated Parmesan cheese

**Directions:**

Combine olive oil, paprika, salt, pepper and garlic powder together. Toss in the cauliflower florets and place in a baking dish in one layer. Bake in a preheated to 350 F oven for 20 minutes. Take out of the oven, stir, and sprinkle with Parmesan cheese. Bake for 5 minutes more or until golden.

## Easy Okra and Tomato Casserole

**Serves: 4**

**Prep time: 25 min**

**Ingredients:**

1 lb okra, trimmed

3 tomatoes, cut into wedges

3 garlic cloves, chopped

1 cup fresh parsley leaves, finely cut

3 tbsp extra virgin olive oil

1 tsp salt

black pepper, to taste

**Directions:**

In a deep ovenproof baking dish, combine okra, sliced tomatoes, olive oil and garlic. Add in salt and black pepper to taste, and toss to combine. Bake in a preheated to 350 F oven for 45 minutes, or until the okra is tender. Sprinkle with parsley and serve.

## Avocado and Feta Toast with Poached Eggs

**Serves: 4**

**Prep time: 5 min**

**Ingredients:**

1 avocado, peeled and chopped

½ cup feta cheese, crumbled

2 tbsp chopped fresh mint

1 tsp lime juice

½ tsp cumin

4 thick slices rye bread, lightly toasted

4 poached eggs

**Directions:**

Mash avocados with a fork until almost smooth. Add the feta, fresh mint, lime juice and cumin. Season with salt and pepper to taste. Stir to combine.

Toast 4 slices of rye bread until golden. Spoon 1/4 of the avocado mixture onto each slice of bread. Top with a poached egg and serve immediately.

## Quick Vegetable Scramble

**Serves: 4**

**Prep time: 10 min**

**Ingredients:**

1/2 small onion, chopped

2 tomatoes, diced

1/4 cup fresh peas

6 eggs

10 oz feta cheese, crumbled

4 tbsp extra virgin olive oil

black pepper, to taste

salt, to taste

**Directions:**

In a large pan sauté onion over medium heat for 1-2 minutes, stirring. Add in tomatoes and peas and simmer until the peas are soft and the mixture is almost dry. Add in feta cheese and eggs, stir, and cook until well mixed and not too liquid.

Season with black pepper and serve.

## Raisin Quinoa Breakfast

**Serves: 4**

**Prep time: 15 min**

**Ingredients:**

1 cup quinoa

2 cups milk

2 tbsp walnuts, crushed

2 tbsp raisins

2 tbsp dried cranberries

2-3 tbsp honey, optional

½ tsp vanilla extract

1 tbsp chia seeds

**Directions:**

Rinse quinoa with cold water and drain. Place milk and quinoa into a saucepan and bring to a boil. Add vanilla. Reduce heat to low and simmer for about 15 minutes stirring from time to time.

Set aside to cool then serve in a bowl, topped with honey, chia seeds, raisins, cranberries and crushed walnuts.

## Hearty Quinoa and Spinach Breakfast Casserole

**Serves: 4**

**Prep time: 30 min**

**Ingredients:**

1 cup cooked quinoa

3-4 spring onions, finely chopped

5 oz frozen chopped spinach, thawed and squeezed dry

½ zucchini, peeled and shredded

5 eggs

1/2 cup milk

4 tbsp extra virgin olive oil

salt and black pepper, to taste

1 cup cheddar cheese, grated

**Directions:**

In a large bowl combine eggs, milk, salt and pepper.

In a deep casserole dish heat the olive oil. Cook the onions, zucchini and spinach, stirring constantly, until lightly cooked. Add in the quinoa and combine everything well. Pour the egg mixture over and then top with cheddar cheese.

Bake in a preheated to 350 F oven for 20 minutes.

## Quick Quinoa Vegetable Scramble

**Serves: 4**

**Prep time: 10 min**

**Ingredients:**

1/2 cup cooked quinoa

1/2 small onion, chopped

2 tomatoes, diced

1 large red pepper, chopped

5 eggs

1/2 cup crumbled feta

4 tbsp extra virgin olive oil

black pepper, to taste

salt, to taste

**Directions:**

In a large pan, sauté onion over medium heat for 1-2 minutes, stirring. Add in tomatoes and red pepper and cook until the mixture is almost dry.

Stir in quinoa, feta and eggs and cook until well mixed and not too liquid.

Season with black pepper and serve.

## Avocado and Pumpkin Muffins

**Serves: 13-14**

**Prep time: 20 min**

**Ingredients:**

1/2 cup mashed avocado

11/2 cup pumpkin puree

2 large eggs

2 cups whole wheat flour

2/3 cup honey

1 tsp baking soda

1 tsp salt

1 tsp cinnamon

1 tsp vanilla extract

1/2 cup walnuts, coarsely chopped

**Directions:**

Preheat oven to 375 F. Grease a muffin tin or line with paper cups.

In a large bowl, mix avocado, pumpkin, eggs and honey. In a separate bowl, whisk flour, baking soda, cinnamon, vanilla and salt. Combine with avocado mixture; do not over-mix. Stir in walnuts.

Spoon batter into prepared muffin tin; bake for 15-18 minutes or until tops start to brown and a toothpick inserted into a muffin comes out clean.

## Blueberry Yogurt Dessert

**Serves 6**

**Prep time: 15 min**

**Ingredients:**

2 cups fresh blueberries

2 tbsp honey

1/2 cup soup cream

3 cups Greek yogurt, strained

1 tsp vanilla extract

**Directions:**

Strain the yogurt in a piece of cheesecloth or a clean white dishtowel. You can suspend it over a bowl or the sink overnight.

In a large bowl, whisk the cream and honey. Add the strained yogurt and vanilla and beat until medium peaks form and the mixture is creamy and thick.

Gently fold half the fresh blueberries into the yogurt mixture until just barely combined, with streaks remaining. Divide dessert among 6 glass bowls, top with fresh blueberries and serve.

## Fresh Strawberries in Mascarpone and Rose Water

**Serves 4**

**Prep time: 5 min**

**Ingredients:**

3 cups strawberries, washed

1 cup mascarpone cheese

1/2 teaspoon rose water

1/2 teaspoon vanilla extract

1/4 cup honey

**Directions:**

In a bowl, combine together the mascarpone cheese, honey, rose water and vanilla. Divide the strawberries into 4 dessert bowls. Top with two dollops of the mascarpone mixture and serve.

## FREE BONUS RECIPES: 10 Clean Eating Quinoa Recipes Anyone Will Love!

## Apricot Chicken with Almonds and Quinoa

**Serves: 4**

**Prep time: 45 min**

**Ingredients:**

2 lb boneless chicken breasts or thighs, cut in 1-2 inch pieces

1 lb apricots, roughly chopped, pits removed and discarded

1 cup orange juice

1 cup quinoa, rinsed

1/4 cup blanched almonds

2 cups homemade chicken broth

1 tsp ground cinnamon

1 tsp turmeric

salt and black pepper, to taste

**Directions:**

In a deep pan, combine orange juice with apricots, almonds, turmeric and cinnamon. Bring to a boil then reduce heat to medium-low and boil for 10 minutes or until the liquid is reduced by half.

Add in the chicken and chicken broth and bring to a boil. Stir in quinoa and simmer for 35 minutes or until cooked through.

Season to taste with salt and pepper to taste and serve.

## Chicken Stew with Sweet Potatoes and Quinoa

**Serves: 4**

**Prep time: 20 min**

**Ingredients:**

2 lb boneless chicken thighs

2 lb sweet potatoes, peeled and cut into chunks

1 small onion, chopped

2-3 garlic cloves

1 cup quinoa, rinsed

1 cup homemade chicken broth or water

1 can crushed tomatoes

1 cup roasted peanuts

1 tsp ground ginger

1 tsp ground coriander

salt and black pepper, to taste

**Directions:**

Heat the vegetable oil in a large soup pot set over medium-high heat. Salt the chicken pieces well, pat them dry and brown them in the oil.

Add in the onions, garlic and ginger and sauté for 1-2 minutes, stirring often.

Stir in the chicken broth, tomatoes, sweet potatoes, peanuts, sugar, coriander and bring to a boil. Simmer for 15 minutes then add quinoa and cook for 15 minutes more or until cooked through.

Season to taste with salt and pepper to taste, and serve.

## Lazy Mustard Chicken with Quinoa

**Serves: 4**

**Prep time: 45 min**

**Ingredients:**

2 lb chicken thighs

2 garlic cloves, crushed

1/2 cup quinoa, rinsed

1 cup water

1/4 to 1/3 cup Dijon mustard

2 tbsp honey

1 tsp dried rosemary

2 tbsp extra virgin olive oil

salt and pepper, to taste

**Directions:**

Gently heat the olive oil in a shallow casserole dish over medium-low heat and sauté the garlic for about a minute, stirring.

In a medium bowl, whisk together the mustard, water, honey and dried rosemary.

Season the chicken pieces with salt and black pepper to taste and lay them skin-side up. Spoon the honey mustard sauce over the chicken.

Bake in a preheated to 350 F oven for 30 minutes. Add in quinoa, stir, and bake until the chicken is cooked through, about 15 more minutes.

## Beef with Quinoa and Melting Onions

**Serves: 6**

**Prep time: 120 min**

**Ingredients:**

2 lb stewing beef

1 cup quinoa, rinsed

4 large onions, sliced

3 garlic cloves, chopped

1 bay leaf

2 cups water

4 tbsp extra virgin olive oil

1 tsp cinnamon

1/2 tsp ginger powder

salt and black pepper, to taste

**Directions:**

Heat olive oil in a large saucepan and brown the beef. Add in the onions and garlic and sauté for 2-3 minutes, stirring.

Add in cinnamon, ginger, the bay leaf, black pepper and water. Bring to a boil. Reduce heat to low, cover, and simmer for about 90 minutes, stirring occasionally. When the beef is almost done, add in quinoa, stir and simmer for 20 minutes more.

## Chicken, Quinoa and Cabbage Casserole

**Serves: 4-5**

**Prep time: 50 min**

**Ingredients:**

1 lb ground chicken meat

1 cup quinoa, rinsed

1/2 cabbage, shredded

1/2 onion, chopped

2 leeks, white part only, chopped

1 tomato, diced

1 tbsp paprika

1/2 tsp cumin

½ tsp black pepper

4 tbsp extra virgin olive oil

salt, to taste

**Directions:**

In a deep saucepan, sauté the onion and leeks in olive oil until tender. Add in the ground chicken, quinoa, tomato, paprika, cumin, salt and black pepper. Stir very well.

Place shredded cabbage on the bottom of an ovenproof baking dish. Cover with beef and quinoa mixture. Cover with a lid or aluminum foil and bake at 325 F for 40 minutes.

## Citrus Pork with Quinoa

**Serves 5-6**

**Prep time: 80 min**

**Ingredients:**

2 lb pork shoulder, cut into 1 inch chunks

1 cup quinoa, rinsed

1 cup orange juice

1 cup water

1 large carrot, chopped

6-7 spring onions, finely cut

1-2 garlic cloves, chopped

1 tbsp lemon zest

1/2 tsp cumin

3 tbsp extra virgin olive oil

**Directions:**

Heat the olive oil in a large skillet over medium-high heat. Working in batches, brown the pieces of pork shoulder.

Add in the carrots, garlic, lemon zest, cumin, salt and black pepper to taste. Stir, and cook for 1-2 minutes, stirring.

Add the orange juice and water, bring to a simmer and cook for 40 minutes.

Stir in quinoa and spring onions and cook for 15 minutes more.

## Spicy Pork Stew with Leeks and Quinoa

**Serves 5-6**

**Prep time: 80 min**

**Ingredients:**

2 lb pork shoulder, cut into 1 inch chunks

1 cup quinoa, rinsed

1 lb leeks, cut

1 large carrot, chopped

1 red pepper, cut

4-5 garlic cloves, chopped

1 tbsp paprika

1 tsp hot paprika

3 tbsp extra virgin olive oil

2 tbsp tomato paste, dissolved in 1/3 cup water

**Directions:**

Heat the olive oil in a large pot over medium-high heat. Working in batches, brown the pieces of pork shoulder.

Add in the carrot, pepper, leeks, garlic, salt, black pepper to taste and paprika. Stir, and add the tomato paste. Bring to a simmer and cook for one hour.

Stir in quinoa and cook for 15 minutes more.

## Comforting Lamb and Quinoa Shepherd's Stew

**Serves: 4-5**

**Prep time: 60 min**

**Ingredients:**

4 shoulder lamb chops, de-boned and cubed

1 cup quinoa

1 ½ cups water

1 onion, finely cut

2 garlic cloves, chopped

2 red peppers, chopped

1 carrot, cut into bite size pieces

1 turnip, cut into bite size pieces

6-7 white mushrooms, chopped

1-2 tomatoes, diced

2 tbsp extra virgin olive oil

1 tbsp paprika

1 bay leaf

1 tbsp thyme

*Directions:*

Wash quinoa very well, drain and set aside.

In a large soup pot or casserole dish, heat the oil over medium heat and brown the meat for 8-10 minutes. Add the onion, bell peppers and garlic and cook until softened, about 3 minutes.

Stir in paprika, the bay leaf and thyme. Add the other vegetables and mushrooms and cook for 1-2 minutes, stirring. Add in the water, bring to the boil and simmer for 30 minutes. Stir in the quinoa and simmer for 15 minutes more.

## Tuna and Quinoa Patties

**Serves: 7**

**Prep time: 20-30 min**

**Ingredients:**

2 6 oz cans tuna

1/2 cup cooked quinoa

1 large egg

1 tbsp Dijon mustard

2 tbsp lemon juice

2-3 spring onions, finely chopped

½ cup fresh parsley, finely chopped

1/4 cup extra virgin olive oil

1 tsp salt

black pepper, to taste

**Directions:**

In a medium bowl, mix together the tuna, mustard, quinoa, lemon juice, spring onions, parsley, and salt. Add in freshly ground black pepper and the egg.

Using your hands, form batter into burgers. Bake in a preheated to 375F oven for 7-8 minutes or until golden.

## Vegetable Quinoa Stew

**Serves: 4-5**

**Prep time: 25 min**

**Ingredients:**

1 cup quinoa

1 ½ cup water

1 onion, finely cut

2 red bell peppers, chopped

1 zucchini, peeled and chopped

1 cup fresh green peas

5-6 green beans

1 tomato, chopped

1 potato, peeled and diced

2 garlic cloves, chopped

1 tbsp paprika

3 tbsp extra virgin olive oil

salt, to taste

½ cup fresh dill, finely cut, to serve

**Directions:**

Rinse the quinoa very well in a sieve under running water and set aside to drain.

Heat olive oil in large saucepan over medium-high heat. Add in the onion and sauté for 1-2 minutes. Add the garlic, paprika, bell pepper, green peas, green beans and zucchini.

Cook, stirring occasionally, for 5 minutes then add the tomato, the potato, and the water.

Bring to the boil and add in quinoa. Stir, cover, and cook for 20 minutes. Season with salt to taste and serve sprinkled with dill.

## About the Author

Alissa Grey is a fitness and nutrition enthusiast who loves to teach people about losing weight and feeling better about themselves. She lives in a small French village in the foothills of a beautiful mountain range with her husband, three teenage kids, two free spirited dogs, and various other animals.

Alissa is incredibly lucky to be able to cook and eat natural foods, mostly grown nearby, something she's done since she was a teenager. She enjoys yoga, running, reading, hanging out with her family, and growing organic vegetables and herbs.

Printed in Great Britain
by Amazon

50644946R00085